POSTURING TOWARDS WHOLENESS

Thomas L. Lenz

Posturing Towards Wholeness

Our Radical Way Forward to Living Well as Healthcare Professionals

Posturing Towards Wholeness: Our Radical Way Forward to Living Well as Healthcare Professionals

By: Thomas L. Lenz

Copyright © 2023 Thomas L. Lenz

This work is licensed under a Standard Copyright License. All rights reserved. This book or any portion thereof may not be reproduced or used in any manner whatsoever without the express written permission of the author except for the use of brief quotations in a book review or scholarly journal.

Lulu Press, Inc. Morrisville, North Carolina

ISBN: 978-1-312-75109-5

Printed in the United States of America

Disclaimer: Because of the dynamic nature of the internet, any web addresses or links contained in this book may have changed since the publication and may no longer be valid. The views expressed in this work are solely those of the author and do not necessarily reflect the views of the publisher.

CONTENTS

Preface 9

Chapter 1. Living Well as Healthcare Professionals 13
    Stress Prevalence and the Influence of a Pandemic 15
    Pathophysiology of the Stress Effect 16
    Perception is Key 18

Chapter 2. Forward 21
    Our Evolution Forward 21
    Recognizing Patterns Towards (and Against) Wholeness 23

Chapter 3. Radical Way 27
    The Radical Way Isn't Radical at All 27
    Radical Wholeness 29

Chapter 4. Our 31
    Relationality 32
    The Science of Connection and Relationship 33
        The Big Bang Theory 34
        The Iron Story 35
        Quantum Physics 36
        Electromagnetic Fields of Energy 36
        Social Networks and Connectedness 38
        The Harvard Study of Adult Development 39
    Compassionate Care Connection 39

Chapter 5. Wholeness 41
    True Self and Separate Self 42
    Tinkering and Transformation 44
    Oneing and Woning 45
    Wholeness in Healthcare 46

Chapter 6. Towards 49
    Intentionality 49
    Discovering What is Ours To Do 50

Chapter 7. Posturing 53
    Contemplation in Practice 54
    Posturing Practice 55
        The Ignatian Daily Examen 56
        The Centering Prayer 57
        The Welcoming Prayer 58
    Posturing as a Healthcare Professional 60

Emerging Thoughts 63

References 67

PREFACE

I once read a quote many years back that said, "How you do anything is how you do everything." I cannot remember where I originally read this, but I have read it many times since. This saying seems to resonate with me because it denotes an underlying quality of character that leads toward consistent action regardless of setting or context. I also like it because it's just plain 'ol good wisdom, such as my dad used to pass along to me and that I try to pass along to my own children. I believe the wisdom in this quote says something about the topic we are about to dive into.

Over the past few decades, a concerning trend among healthcare professionals points to a rise in the symptoms of burnout. The term burnout was first used in a publication by Hubert Freudenberger in 1974.[1] Dr. Freudenberger was a clinical psychologist and used burnout to describe an unreasonable demand for energy and other personal resources. He described the symptoms of burnout to be malaise, fatigue, frustration, cynicism, and inefficacy. Today, burnout is a word frequently used by many, and within many professions, to describe poor work-life balance and the outcomes of feeling overworked and overwhelmed. An official measurement tool for burnout was first published in 1981 by Christina Maslach called The Maslach Burnout Inventory.[2] This widely accepted and validated scale measures burnout on the characteristics of emotional exhaustion, depersonalization (the inability to recognize the humanness in others), and a diminished sense of personal accomplishment.

Around 2010, amid growing concern for burnout in physicians, researchers from the American Medical Association, The Mayo Clinic, and Stanford University began tracking the prevalence of burnout.[3] Collectively, these studies found that in 2011 over 45% of physicians practicing in the United States were experiencing burnout. This prevalence rose to over 54% in 2014 but then dipped in

2017 and 2020 (pre-pandemic) to levels of 44% and 38%, respectively. However, with the onset of COVID-19, the prevalence of burnout among American physicians sharply rose to nearly 63% in 2021. This can be compared to an overall burnout rate of 52% that same year among all healthcare providers combined.[4] These numbers demonstrate why there is a growing concern about this condition, as the healthcare industry is the largest U.S. employer, with over 22 million workers.[5]

The impact of burnout among healthcare professionals and the healthcare system is extraordinary. Research shows that, specifically among physicians, burnout leads to two times higher odds of making medical errors.[6] It also costs the healthcare industry $12 billion annually due to the high rate of physician turnover alone.[7-10] Most concerning, however, is that physicians who experience burnout have a suicide rate over twice that of the general population (28 to 40 vs. 12 per 100,000 people).[11] The situation of burnout in the U.S. healthcare system is so significant that the National Academy of Medicine considers it to be a public health problem.[12]

Much has been written lately about what can be done to turn the tide of the growing burnout epidemic. But one of the most convincing solutions to this issue may come as a surprise to some. In a recent book called *Compassionomics,* authors Dr. Stephen Trzeciak and Dr. Anthony Mazzarelli provide a rigorous systematic review of the published literature that convincingly shows that healthcare providers who offer greater compassion to patients, coworkers, and themselves not only provide better care to patients but experience less burnout themselves.[13] Hundreds of studies were reviewed throughout the book to show that offering patients more meaningful connections through compassionate practices significantly improves physiological and psychological outcomes, motivates patients to adhere to medication therapy and self-care practices, and also decreases overall healthcare costs. What is surprising, however, is that giving more compassion to others also shows a scientific and statistically significant inverse relationship with burnout. In other words, healthcare providers who give the most compassion experience the least amount of burnout. And the opposite is also true. Healthcare providers who give the least compassion to their patients experience the greatest amount of burnout. And as a side note, in case you were wondering, the average amount of extra time it takes for a healthcare provider to give high-level compassion to patients is, on average, an extra 40 seconds compared to care that does not deliver high compassion.[13]

Why should it be surprising that having a greater connection with others improves the health of both the receiver and the giver? And why should it be surprising that the notion of relationship may be a foundational and fundamental part of the care we provide to others? Hopefully, we can answer these important questions as we make our way through this book. The purpose, then, of this book is not to review the scientific data related to compassionate care. Rather, the purpose here is to dive in deeper as to why and how giving compassion to others and making more meaningful connections leads to a life of living well for others and ourselves. The compassion we offer to others is an extension of ourselves, a relational flow from one person to another if you will. But this flow moves in two directions, not just from the giver to the receiver but also from the receiver back again to the giver. This relational exchange will provide the basis of our conversations throughout the book and will hopefully lead to more insight as to why our connection to others and the compassion we provide is critical to living well.

BOOK PRESENTATION STRATEGY

It may be unconventional, but the presentation strategy of the material for this book seems to make the most sense by going backward. By that, I mean the words within the book title, *Posturing Towards Wholeness: Our Radical Way Forward to Living Well as Healthcare Professionals,* will make up the seven chapter titles and proceed in reverse order, starting with *Chapter 1: Living Well as Healthcare Professionals.* This chapter lays a foundation of sorts by reviewing our current state of stress and connecting the pathophysiology and side effects of stress on the body, mind, and emotional centers. It also briefly discusses our movements towards stress as Americans and how we have adopted it as an everyday way of life, particularly within the healthcare setting. *Chapter Two: Forward,* reviews the current models we use to minimize stress from the perspective of their abilities to move us forward toward transformation rather than simply trying to cope with stress. This chapter also introduces the concept of wholeness that is built upon throughout the remainder of the book. *Chapter Three: Radical Way,* gets to the fundamental nature of stress, fatigue, and burnout and relates it to wholeness as the center of our humanness. *Chapter Four: Our,* begins with the notion that relationality is fundamental to well-being. It reviews the scientific evidence that connects us as humans to all that is, such that our well-being is connected and dependent upon the well-being of all else, including each other. *Chapter Five: Wholeness,* makes the argument that when we talk about health and wellness, we are really talking about wholeness. It brings forward the concepts of relationality and unity to explore a way of life rooted in non-dual consciousness that leads to transformation. *Chapter Six: Towards,* discusses the greater importance of intentionality in our movement toward transformation and wholeness as opposed to the goal of achievement that much of our healthcare system and society emphasizes. *Chapter Seven: Posturing,* is the "how to" part of the book. This chapter offers examples of the countless ways we can put ourselves in a position of connection with others, or a relational exchange, as we will call it, as we move toward transformation and wholeness.

The concepts discussed throughout this book are not new because the importance of relationships has been talked about for millennia. However, they are rarely discussed with any kind of seriousness within the healthcare system, as crazy as that may seem. If we want to change the increasing tide of healthcare provider burnout, it may be time for us to more fully understand the importance that relationality plays within the system, but most importantly, within those who come to the system for care and those who provide it.

Chapter 1

LIVING WELL AS HEALTHCARE PROFESSIONALS

"Be kind, for everyone you meet is fighting a hard battle."
-Unknown

We often get consumed by our own story in a way that doesn't allow us to see that of others. The quote above reminds us that we have a shared experience in this life that requires us to transcend our individual struggles and recognize that life is not perfect for other people, the same as it is not for us. The author of the quote takes this notion further, however, and suggests that we should act too—as in "be kind." The advice may seem simple at first glance, but it is profound when we take a second look. How often are we unable to recognize the pain and suffering in others (at work and at home) because we are only consumed with our own? Are there shared experiences that, if addressed on both the personal and community levels, can reduce the stress of the "hard battle" regardless of context?

As presented in the *Preface*, the focus of this book is on our movement toward wholeness and a life of living well as healthcare professionals. Living well can mean many things, but what it means in the context of wholeness will hopefully become clearer as this book progresses. A good place to begin our understanding of living well might be to look at the opposite, however. What does "un-well" look like? And in particular, what does it look like in the life of a healthcare professional? What are some indicators that point to the "hard battle," as the quote says, that most healthcare providers seem to be fighting? Some of these indicators include the prevalence of stress, fatigue, and burnout.

Stress is not a new concept. Naturally, some stress is necessary to motivate us for daily life. Our urges to avoid danger, find food, and get a job to pay for life's necessities are all examples of necessary stress. Naming these urges as stress began in the 1920s when stress was used to describe the strain on physical objects by external forces.[14] Hans Selye (1907-1982), the founder of the stress theory, was the first to use the term stress to describe the physiological responses of the body toward stress. The term was later used to describe the psychological and emotional strain of both external and internal forces.[14]

Although the initial research on stress described short-term physiological adaptations to stress, most of the research over the past 100 years has come to study the long-term manifestations of stress. These long-term or prolonged stress events have come to be known collectively as chronic stress and account for most of the stress events experienced by people today.[15] In general, it is estimated that about 55% of Americans experience daily stress.[16] More specifically, however, It is reported that 93% of healthcare providers experience daily stress.[17] The stressors (the events, forces, or conditions that result in physical or psychological stress) in our society at large are abundant. They include poverty, chronic illness, dysfunctional personal relationships, loneliness, feeling out of control with life, political dysfunction, and a pandemic, to name a few. For healthcare providers, sources of stress also come from long work hours, rotating and irregular work shifts, intense and emotional labor, exposure to human suffering and death, increased risk of exposure to disease and violence, feeling that there isn't enough time in the day to meet workloads, over-interaction with technology like the electronic medical record system, and feeling the burden of non-patient facing responsibilities such as insurance coverage issues in addition to the stressors of the general population.[17]

Related to stress, other terms are now being used to describe the outcomes of psychological and physiological symptoms resulting from stressors such as fatigue and burnout. Fatigue has been described by the National Institute for Occupational Safety and Health (NIOSH) as "a feeling of weariness, tiredness, or lack of energy."[18] Others have described fatigue with similar terms because of prolonged physical and mental work, extended periods of anxiety, exposure to a harsh environment, and/or a loss of sleep.[19] Fatigue has been shown to be a major contributor to impaired alertness and performance, a leading cause of dangerous errors, and a factor in decreased quality of life.[19]

Likewise, burnout has been a term used to describe the long-term symptoms of chronic stress. Burnout, as defined by the American Psychological Association, is "physical, emotional, or mental exhaustion accompanied by decreased motivation, lower performance, and negative attitudes towards oneself and others."[20] Healthcare professionals such as physicians, nurses, and emergency medical technicians have identified symptoms such as emotional exhaustion, depersonalization, and a lack of a sense of personal accomplishment to describe burnout.[21]

STRESS PREVALENCE AND THE INFLUENCE OF A PANDEMIC

Regardless of terminology, experiencing stress in both short and long-term forms is part of the human experience. As we will briefly review in the next section of this chapter, we have adapted to external stressors since the beginning of our evolution. To think that stress is not part of life would be the same as thinking we do not need food to eat. We need both food and stress to survive. However, too much of a good thing has a way of creating negative consequences— as is the case for stress (and food). General population data in the United States shows that prior to the COVID-19 pandemic, stress affected about 43% of the population and accounted for about 80% of all primary care physician visits.[22,23] In addition, stress is said to be a significant factor in about 85% of all diseases and illnesses.[22,24] These numbers are striking, yet nothing compared to those experienced during the height of the COVID-19 pandemic. Data published by the American Psychological Association in 2021 showed that nearly 70% of Americans experienced increased stress over the course of the pandemic.[25] Additionally, specific segments of the population, such as 79% of Gen Z adults and 74% of Millennials, experienced behavior changes because of the pandemic.[25] Other data sources reported that over half (55%) of the general American adult population reported struggling with the ups and downs of the pandemic.[26] A Work and Well-Being survey administered by the APA during the pandemic revealed that over 70% of Americans experienced work-related stress, with three in five workers reporting negative stress-related symptoms such as physical fatigue (44%), lack of interest, motivation, or energy (26%), lack of effort at work (19%), cognitive weariness (36%), and emotional exhaustion (32%).[27]

PATHOPHYSIOLOGY OF THE STRESS EFFECT

Many have explained the historical and evolutionary nature of the human stress response.[22,28,29] It has been good and necessary for human survival to avoid and escape from danger, find food and shelter, and meet the needs that are fundamental to survival. However, as it is often cited, our modern-day culture does not typically require us to avoid predatory animals or act as hunters and gathers to obtain our daily nutritional needs. But many aspects of our physiology continue to respond similarly as our ancient ancestors did to the stressor of modern-day living. The major difference, however, is that the stressors of our ancestors were largely short-term, whereas today, they persist for long periods of time. The pathophysiology of the stress response system is complex, and we will not be covering it in any great detail here because it can be better understood elsewhere.[22,28,29] However, it is worth a brief overview to contextualize our conversation on what it means to live well.

In general terms, the complex physiological stress response is triggered when we experience an external event and/or when we replay a past event in our minds. We perceive the event to be positive or negative, and this perception triggers a physiological response based on our perception. A negatively perceived event or memory will cause our body to respond differently than a positive event or memory. The physical mechanism that controls our body's response to a negative event or memory is referred to as the hypothalamus-pituitary-adrenal (HPA) system.[22] When a negative event is perceived, the hypothalamic region of the brain releases a hormone called corticotropin-releasing hormone (CRH). The CRH then stimulates the pituitary gland causing the release of adrenocorticotropin (ACTH) which in turn causes the adrenal glands to produce and release epinephrine, norepinephrine, and cortisol—collectively known as stress hormones.

Once the stress hormones become released into the bloodstream, they can induce many physiological reactions that prepare our bodies for fight or flight. For example, stress hormones increase blood and glucose in our muscles, increase heart rate and blood pressure, increase the ability of the heart to pump blood more effectively, and mobilize insulin so our muscular cells can receive the glucose and the energy they need. Additionally, these hormones increase the tension in our muscles, increase our respiratory rate to supply more oxygen to the lungs for circulation to the heart, brain, and muscles, and stimulate our central nervous system to improve reaction time. The short-term effect of this physiological stress response system is marvelous and has served us well as it protected us throughout our human history. These short-term effects have even been shown to help boost our immune system and cognitive function in more recent studies.[22,28,29] However, they have shown the opposite when they remain activated during long-term stress experiences.

It is easy to see how the physiological response to stressors can benefit human life and survival when it occurs in short bursts. But what happens when the stressor does not go away? Rather than the sharp and brief spike in hormone levels, long-term chronic stress results in a low but persistent release of stress hormones over long periods. These long and persistent elevated levels of stress hormones have been observed in chronic stress situations, such as when people experience poverty, racism, sexism, and gender and sexual preference discrimination.[30-33] Other examples of chronic stress that lead to lasting elevated stress hormone release include living with a chronic illness, being a caregiver for someone with a chronic illness or advanced age, working within a dysfunctional environment or institutional system, single parenting, an unstable or negative political climate, and living through a pandemic.[22-34] And specific to healthcare providers, certain groups have been disproportionately impacted by chronic stress, including health workers of color, immigrant health workers, female health workers, low-wage health workers, and health workers in rural and tribal communities.[35]

These low but persistently elevated levels of stress hormones have been shown to have negative health consequences. Within the cardiovascular system, for example, persistent increases in blood pressure increase the risks of heart attack, stroke, and heart failure.[35] In the endocrine system, dysfunctional insulin and glucose metabolism increase the risk for obesity and type 2 diabetes. The nervous system can negatively affect the gastrointestinal system causing stomach and bowel pain, discomfort, bloating, constipation, diarrhea, gas production, and damage to the good bacteria needed for digestion.[22] Additionally, the nervous system influences the immune system to lower the ability to fight infection and other nervous system functions such as mental clarity, critical thinking skills, and decision-making. Less specific to certain body systems, long-term elevated stress hormones lead to anxiety and worry, decreased energy and motivation, increased irritability and anger, and diminished quality and quantity of sleep.[22]

PERCEPTION IS KEY

After reviewing the pathophysiology of stress and the many illnesses that can result, it is easy to see the connections between chronic stress and chronic illness. The reason it seems necessary to review the physiological stress response system and its connection to chronic illness is an often under-discussed aspect of what actually triggers the stress response system. *The perception of an event or memory is the trigger for the stress response system rather than the event itself.* Studies have shown that HPA activity is not consistent across all people and not even between people experiencing the same stressor.[24] Research shows that two people experiencing the same stressor can have differing levels of HPA activity. One person may have high HPA activity leading to the production of stress hormones, while the other may have low levels of HPA activity leading to little or no stress hormone activity. Specific short-term examples of stressors include being late to an appointment or when trying to meet a tight deadline at work. Long-term examples include caring for an elderly parent or living with a low income. The research shows that the HPA activity is due to each person's unique and individual perception of the stressor more than the stressor itself. Therefore, it may be more accurate to say that the stressor and how the stressor is perceived are both important considerations when developing strategies to mitigate chronic stress.

It is worth noting that although the individual perception of a stressful event is a major contributor to the stimulation of the stress response system, this should in no way minimize how one individual perceives an event compared to another. In other words, if two people experience the exact same stressor and one perceives it as significant and the other does not, this does not mean that each should be judged differently. Often people who perceive stressors as significant are treated as if they should "be stronger" or should "tighten up their bootstraps." They are often treated as if they are somehow weak and less than others who seem to be able to "handle" the stress. This is a critical error in judgment. One person's perception is their reality and if we are to move forward with mitigating the prevalence of chronic stress and burnout, then we need to set aside our impulse to judge the quality and character of others simply based on how they perceive stressful events. This is especially true within the healthcare system.

One of the great stressors for people today is their inability to feel in control of the experiences of day-to-day life. If it is true that our perception of a stressor plays a major role in our personal health, then this is a reason for hope, and we may have more control than we realize. This is an important concept and one that will be addressed later as it gives great justification for a new path forward toward living well as healthcare professionals. Perhaps this new path forward is one that incorporates both the necessary work needed to change the root cause of the stressor and a change in our perception of the stressor itself. In other words, a new definition of living well may include the ability to hold both at the same time. Changing our perception to hold the tension of both can be a place for transformation and an opening to a greater depth dimension and meaning to living well. We will continue to build on this concept as we make our way through the chapters ahead.

Chapter 2

FORWARD

"Evolution is an unfolding of consciousness."
-Pierre Teilhard de Chardin, SJ

The life we live and our passage through time is more than simply the months and years passing by. It is a movement forward and towards continual evolution. As the Jesuit Catholic priest, mystic, and evolutionary biologist Pierre Teilhard de Chardin (1881-1955) wrote about so often, we are individually and collectively part of an evolutionary process that moves us towards something—which he called The Omega.[36] This continual evolution and unfolding of the cosmos and all its parts move towards an ever-increasing awareness of ourselves and of the whole. We are both whole and simultaneously part of the larger whole. This realization becomes clearer with our continual movements toward a greater depth dimension—toward the real Living Well.

OUR EVOLUTION FORWARD

Our forward evolution may be better understood with a second look at our current health and wellness practices. It can be said that our methods and ideas about health and wellness have been good and necessary in many ways. After all, there is a mountain of scientific evidence to support healthy lifestyle behaviors and the positive changes they can make to human physiology. Many people have benefited greatly from research and innovative health and wellness methods over the past several decades. But, regardless of the interventions, we still seem to be struggling. The prevalence of obesity and diabetes continues to rise, and as discussed in the previous chapter, we struggle greatly with stress. Could it be that we are fundamentally wrong in how we see the core issues related to health and wellness? Could our biomedical and reductionistic philosophy of medicine be the rate limiter to greater health when it was designed to be the opposite? As Teilhard has emphasized, humanity and everything else in the cosmos are dynamically evolving toward something greater. It is time for our health and wellness practices to become conscious of our evolution and our movement toward [this] something greater.

Much of our current health and wellness system is focused on individualism rather than including the individual and the community as part of the same whole. In many cases, patients and healthcare providers alike are expected to fix their own health problems. Take, for example, burnout in healthcare. The current system emphasizes a set of individually focused plans rather than modifying individual behaviors at the same time that the larger community modifies the structural influences of the system. Our previous strategies of only focusing on the individual person's side of the equation have blunted our potential for greater health and wellness. Our obsession with individualism combined with our lack of interest in the relationship that each person has with each other and the greater whole of the community has led us down a path of illness that encourages stress and promotes the notion that resiliency is solely the individual's responsibility without connection to the whole of society. If we take a deeper look into the current strategies we implement for stress management, we can see that they are good but perhaps not going far enough to make a difference at a fundamental level.

We place a great deal of emphasis and attention on the "thinking mind" in our current stress management strategies. In other words, the psychological aspects of stress and how we can reframe our thinking minds have gotten most of the attention as the primary method of stress relief. Strategies such as changing our mindset, positive psychology, cognitive restructuring, and the like have all been good and effective therapeutic strategies.[37,38] However, focusing solely on the mind doesn't seem to capture the whole essence of the person or address the origin of the stressor. Addressing both the structurally related issues (i.e., cultural norms within the healthcare system) and modifications at the personal level (perceiving the stressor as a threat) may be a more effective strategy. Additionally, strategies that include psychological strategies *and* those that lead us towards greater awareness, wholeness, and transformation incorporate our many ways of knowing—not just that of our cognitive minds.

RECOGNIZING PATTERNS TOWARDS (AND AGAINST) WHOLENESS

Much has been written about the influence that our society has on our health and wellness. In my book, *Chronically American*, I summarized the work of anthropologists, historians, philosophers, scientists, clinicians, and others to show the connections between our American way of life and our ever-increasing prevalence of chronic illness.[39] The Modern Era began in Europe in the 1500s and greatly influenced the birth, growth, and attitudes of our American culture. Modernity emphasized the importance of achievement, intellectual reasoning, a reliance on knowledge from science, a focus on individualism and self-orientation (over collectivism), and the belief in perfectibility. Then, beginning in the late 20th Century, the Post-Modern Era began to emerge, but out of notions of skepticism and suspicion. While modernists championed clarity and simplicity, post-modernism embraced complex and often contradictory layers of meaning. Key features of the Post-Modern Era include globalization, the media, a fragmented world (due to social change), consumerism with individual freedom to choose one's lifestyle, cultural diversity, and using human identity as a social construct. Additionally, post-modernism emphasizes pluralism and relativism while at the same time rejecting certainty about beliefs and absolute value.[40] However, even though we are well on our way to post-modernism, it is important to understand that transitions between major eras are just that, a transition. The ideals of the Modern Era are now blended with those of the Post-Modern Era, and characteristics of both are prominent in our lives today.

Our evolution as a society and culture is neither good nor bad. But it is important to understand that the characteristics that define our cultural movements have a significant influence on our attitudes, norms, and values—and, therefore, on our health and wellness. Once we start recognizing the patterns of our culture that steer us towards our hyper-focus on achievement, for example, we can make the connections between social influences and personal stress. Our continued emphasis on the importance of achievement and the need to accumulate more (e.g., more success, more money, more social media likes, more friends, more accolades, more power, more material goods) often comes with feelings of dissatisfaction. We continually need more to keep the feeling going. This isn't to say that we should abandon our sense of achievement and the competitiveness that moves us in that direction. After all, this is how we make discoveries (especially in science, engineering, and medicine) and work towards a better life. Rather, changing our perception of it as being a threat to our personal identity would be a movement towards—an evolution of greater awareness and consciousness. It is at this intersection that our interpretation of the stressor can change. Our perception of our continual need for achievement as being a threat can change to acceptance. This is not to say that feeling the need for more and more achievement is now acceptable—it's actually the opposite. Acceptance, in this case, is a deeper understanding (i.e., consciousness) of the stress that the healthcare system and society place on us. This deeper understanding and greater level of consciousness can then lead to a diminishing need to have more and, at the same time, know what is ours to do in both our personal and professional lives. This enhanced level of consciousness is a movement towards living well as healthcare professionals in a complex and confusing system and society.

This notion can have great application for healthcare providers at both the personal and system levels. Knowing what is ours to do at a personal level versus a team level versus an organizational level could be of great help when it comes to perceiving stressors. Likewise, increased consciousness at the corporate level can lead an organization to a clarity of knowing how to work effectively, efficiently, and compassionately within a challenging system. Both applications can work independently of each other. But when the personal and organizational levels move in a forward direction of consciousness together, real transformation can happen for the whole. An enhanced level of personal consciousness is a wonderful movement forward for individual health and well-being. But an enhanced collective social consciousness may be even more important and powerful in our movement towards living well as healthcare professionals (and as a society in general).

Teilhard said, "the bloodstream of evolution is love, and it includes union and communion." Our current practices in health and wellness place too much emphasis on the outcomes rather than on the intentionality of the movement forward. This isn't to say that we do not want the best outcomes for our patients. But our movement forward must be one that includes union and communion that moves beyond ourselves. Our movement must be one that includes relationality with a meaningful exchange with others and the world around us. It must transcend our individuality and include the spirit of unity. This is our path toward health and wellness, and we must embrace this first and fundamentally before moving on from our current practices and procedures.

CHAPTER 3

RADICAL WAY

"At the bottom of all reality is always a deep goodness, and you can't get much more radical than that."
-Fr. Richard Rohr, OFM

At the end of the previous chapter, a mention of intentionality was given without a lot of contexts. We will spend a great deal more time on the notion of intentionality in Chapter Six, but this quote from Fr. Richard already gets us part way there. When Fr. Richard says, "At the bottom," he is talking about the absolute foundational level—the source, if you will. An important piece of our movement toward wholeness is a fundamental desire, an authentic intention, for goodness and love. When we have this as our starting place from which to build towards wholeness and living well, then we are starting with fundamental goodness, as Fr. Richard says, which is true Reality.

THE RADICAL WAY ISN'T RADICAL AT ALL

If our current health and wellness methods are not fulfilling in the way we would like, then we need to keep looking. This looking may lead to disappointment in the system and maybe even in ourselves in how we have been doing our business. But eventually, if we move with intentionality towards wholeness, it will result in peace, contentment, and freedom to accept "what is" as part of the evolutionary process and, at the same time, take the necessary steps towards something new. Looking at our current situation in healthcare from a "step back" view allows us to see the whole of the experience more clearly. It makes room for us to look for something more basic, more fundamental, and more meaningful. It allows for something that makes more sense, and not just in our cognitive brain, but in the heart as well.

The use of the term radical in the context of this chapter may be a bit confusing. Our pop culture often uses the term radical to refer to something extreme. But the actual meaning of radical relates to the fundamental nature of something. It comes from the Latin word *radicalis* or to "have roots." For our conversation here, *Our Radical Way Forward* takes the meaning of "a fundamental action" necessary to move towards *Living Well as Healthcare Professionals*.

In the book *Chronically American*, I spend some time discussing the term "lifeworld." Jurgen Habermas, a German sociologist and philosopher, first used the concept of lifeworld. Habermas used lifeworld to describe an individual's [or group's] "taken-for-granted view of the world that provides understanding and meaning to life."[41,42] These taken-for-granted presuppositions exist below conscious awareness and do not always allow us to discern what is meaningful about life. We can easily apply lifeworld to describe common parts of our daily life, such as the pre-packaged, highly processed, and highly sugared foods we find in the supermarket. We can also apply lifeworld to our education system to describe its linear and reductionistic methodologies. In our healthcare system, the lifeworld describes the acceptable yet dysfunctional fee-for-service reimbursement model, our reliance on inefficient levels of communication, and the constant undertones of urgency in non-emergent situations, to name a few. Other lifeworlds exist within the institutions of politics, economics, and government. What we learn from Habermas' work is that social influence can set the norms, attitudes, and practices for the community members rather than the community members setting these values for themselves. As we have discussed in the previous chapter, when cultural norms, attitudes, and practices support personal and collective characteristics such as the need for more money, power, academic degrees, social media responses, and the like as the lifeworld, it can place undue stress on the community and its members. Therefore, when we think about our healthcare system and our health and wellness practices with lifeworld in mind, we can use it to justify the need to consider a new path.

RADICAL WHOLENESS

As we work toward wholeness in this book, it's a good time to introduce it as a radical concept. Wholeness is rooted in our humanness. Wholeness is such a part of our truest selves that we have a deep longing for wholeness—a topic we will dive into further in Chapter Five. If we can connect to this wholeness, both personally and collectively, then our experience of living well may be able to flourish in unexpected ways and lead to transformation.

How do we know that wholeness is fundamental and central to our humanness? As a brief introduction to our next chapter, several indicators are present that point to this belief. Over the past 100 years, the science community has given us great insight into what they believe to be the beginning moments of the cosmos.[43] There is evidence to support the notion that everything we know of in the universe began at a single point in time and is referred to as the Big Bang, which is believed to have occurred about 13.7 billion years ago. Since that moment, all that we know has developed from that singularity. Even if scientists are proven wrong about the timeframe and origin, which is likely, it will not change the fact that everything developed and continues to develop from that singularity. This means everything in the past, present, and future is connected to the singularity. This can only make sense when we look at all that is and ever was through an interconnected and whole perspective. And because this is who we are at a fundamental level, we greatly long to be part of a whole beyond our individual selves. There will be much more to say about this later.

Many other examples of wholeness are present in our lives as well. For example, our bodies are made of many individual parts but naturally act as an interconnected whole. Our body parts cannot exist unless connected to the greater whole. And at the same time, the body is reliant on the individual parts to make it whole. Wholeness can also be thought of in the same way using the examples of an orchestra, band, singing groups, and sports teams. In each of these examples, the whole is greater than the sum of its parts. The experience is almost always better with a group rather than individually. A loss for a sports team doesn't feel quite as bad compared to an individual loss because of the collective experience. And a win almost always feels better when experienced with others compared to an individual experience.

Other day-to-day examples point to the desire to form social communities, work groups, and clubs that gather people together. In all these examples, our connection and desire to be with others are critical to our survival and quality of life, despite our socially influenced lifeworld towards individualism. When we transcend beyond ourselves and toward others, we know it feels good. And when we isolate ourselves and are only consumed with our own personal issues, we know it feels bad and leads to stress, anxiety, and depression.

This concept is particularly poignant in our healthcare system. A lifeworld that only recognizes individual productivity, gains, and losses results in winners and losers and fragmented othering. But a reimagined system that looks towards the collective (system and providers as one whole) could produce better results for all. This may be part of the hidden message in the book *Compassionomics* by Trzeciak and Mazzarelli that was introduced in the *Preface*.[13] When healthcare providers give more compassion to their patients, not only do their patients experience better outcomes, but so do the providers and organization. Giving compassion to others seems to make room for the provider to experience less burnout and greater work satisfaction and for the organization to show a more robust bottom line. This is a movement towards the collective and is an example of how everyone benefits from being part of the same whole.

Our authentic desire and the energy we use to connect with others and the world around us have collectively been described by many simply as love. Wholeness and love are inseparable. In the words of Sr. Ilia Delio, "our challenge today is to trust the power of love at the heart of life, to let ourselves be seized by love, to create and invent ways for love to evolve into a global wholeness of unity, compassion, justice, and peacemaking." At our most fundamental and radical level, love is the foundation. To move closer to living well means we radically start with love.

CHAPTER 4

OUR

"The final end product of this continuous vortex of Exchange, of giving, of receiving, of dynamism, the final product of Exchange is abundance."
-Rev. Cynthia Bourgeault

When I was a young boy, my parents would take my siblings and me to my grandparent's house for dinner on a regular basis. Sometimes there would be more people than just my immediate family members. But no matter how many people were there, my Grandma Alice was always busy in the kitchen preparing more than enough food for everyone. At some point during the meal, someone would always make a comment about how good the food was and especially about the amount of food she cooked and baked for the gathering. Her response was always the same…"I'm just happy we could all be together."

For decades researchers have been trying to find the key aspects of a life well lived. Some have studied the foods we eat, others the activities we do, and still others the locations of where we live, the amount of money we have, the types of careers we give our time to, and on and on. We have studied these aspects of our lives and the way they make us feel happy and grateful and provide a sense of peace, security, and satisfaction. And the data is clear in pointing to one singular aspect—relationships. The relationships we have in our lives appear to be the single most important factor to happiness, well-being, and a life well lived over and above where we live, the amount of money we have, and the types of jobs and titles we achieve.

One aspect of a relationship that helps us to understand our participation in the whole is that of the exchange. It only takes one experience of a loving relationship to understand the importance of the exchange—we give a part of ourselves to another, and that other gives something back to us to receive, and we again return with more giving and more receiving. But what is passed back and forth? The answer is easy, Love! Regardless of whether we are experiencing this love from our parents, a friend, a partner, our pets, or some other aspect of nature, a dynamic exchange of love is taking place. And the reason that this relational exchange makes us feel a greater sense of happiness, joy, freedom, and safety is its rootedness in abundance. The more we give, the more we receive. We cannot say that about any other parts of life that we use to try to make us happy. Love never runs out, there is an endless supply. This aspect of the relational exchange only needs to be experienced once to know that it can be trusted because the source of love is Love itself.

Long before scientific research was published about the importance of relationships, Grandma Alice already knew. The relational exchange of love that we all experienced at those dinner gatherings was the "secret sauce" to the meal. The abundance of food on the table couldn't match the abundance of love given and received by all. I don't think I could ever find a better example of wisdom and truth in any research project I could ever do.

The focus of this chapter is on Grandma Alice's secret sauce. We will spend considerable time looking at a select few important scientific projects that show the importance of relationships within our lives. Even though we don't need scientific proof to tell us when we feel like we are living well, the data and information help us to connect what we feel in our hearts and bodies to that which we comprehend with our minds.

RELATIONALITY

The term relationality seems to be very fitting as we expand our understanding of our connections with others. It describes the exchange that occurs between…well, everything. In a relationship, there are patterns of giving, receiving, and giving back again—an exchange. Holding on, or clinging to what we have, is not part of relationality. Giving away is primary without concern for the questions of "how much?" or "will there be enough left for me?". True relationality involves counter-intuitive giving because there is an understanding and trust that it is rooted in abundance rather than scarcity. Within relationality, there is a sense of peace that there will always be enough.

In the previous chapter, we looked at our cultural evolution as Americans and outlined the individualism-based values that have come to be our lifeworld. It's important to pause here and recognize that these characteristics and attitudes are not bad and are probably even necessary, especially early in life. But they can also be taken too far and to a place where they are projected onto others in a way that says, "I don't need you or anyone else." When we get to this place, we begin to feel the fear of scarcity and the unhealthy competition that is needed so that our personal well (metaphorically speaking) does not run dry of the perception that we have enough fame, glory, attention, and self-worth (i.e., ego). This is not what it means to truly live well. Self-reliance is good, but not at the expense of furthering an unhealthy amount of individualism.

Relationality, on the other hand, focuses on the collective (the union) while also not ignoring the importance of the individual. Relationality promotes personal connections at home, work, play, and with our communities. Relationality also promotes our collective connections with our institutions, such as healthcare, education, politics, and economics. Relationality leads to living well because it works with a foot in both the structural (i.e., social, cultural, economic, and political structures) and the personal responsibility causes of illness and disease. Relationality doesn't choose sides but rather recognizes the need to work with both at the same time.

THE SCIENCE OF CONNECTION AND RELATIONSHIP

When we think about relationships, we most often think about them in the ways we are connected to other people. The word connect comes from the Latin word *conectere*, which means to join together. But, if we are to believe that we are part of a grand wholeness that is beyond our individual selves, then we move to an expanded view of relationships—one that includes all that exists. For the remainder of this book, the meaning of relationship will include not only that which we have with other people but also that which we have with all of nature, with God, and even with ourselves. Our relationship, or better yet, our relationality, includes the Whole of everything, both seen and unseen.

It seems it is difficult for us to believe something unless we have scientific proof through research and data. For some reason, we have difficulty trusting the feelings we encounter from our lived experiences in this world. It makes us feel better if we can validate those feelings with some kind of proof. With this in mind, it is appropriate for us to look at the scientific evidence of our connections to the world around us as a way to prove to ourselves that we really are part of a grand wholeness and that our relationships within the wholeness matter. From that starting point, we can then build upon our thinking-centered way of knowing to a heart-centered way of knowing through contemplative practices-which we will do in the subsequent chapters.

The Big Bang Theory

Most of us learned about the Big Bang Theory in elementary school science classes. The central theme is that everything that we know of within the entire universe came from a single starting point—a massive explosion that put everything we know of into motion. The most recent research estimates that the starting point is believed to be about 13.7 billion years ago.[43] And, as a reference point, our earth is believed to be about 4.54 billion years old. It is likely that these estimations will change as our technology improves and we develop more sophisticated ways of seeing and measuring the universe.

Regardless of the exact age, however, the notion that everything began from a singular moment is important to our thinking mind's understanding of wholeness. Logically we can understand that if everything developed and expanded from a single moment in time, then everything that exists is directly and reductionistically connected back to that singular moment. As hard as it is to imagine, if this is true then each person is in some way connected to every person who is currently living and to everyone who has lived in the past, and to everyone who will live in the future. If that isn't hard enough to wrap our minds around, we are also connected with every animal, every plant, every cloud, and every star that has ever existed or will exist in the future. Each evolving step in this evolutionary process has been dependent upon the previous step. The universe wouldn't be what it is if all the parts were not connected and working together in synergy. Sometimes we may feel like what we are doing doesn't matter much in this world. But our scientific evidence signifies a starting point for which everything has evolved, and every moment within that evolutionary process has a great interdependence upon the last. Therefore, all the parts, as great in number as they are, matter to the whole of everything—including us at this very moment.

Aside from the scientifically based story that can be told about the Big Bang, there is a spiritual story that can be told that is even more compelling. Regardless of religious tradition, if we believe that God set the universe in motion from a singular moment, then God is part of that event and everything that developed from that point forward as well. In other words, God dwells in each of us and in all that exists. God does not just exist outside of us but within us and within everything else, too. In this way, science and spirituality are not separate but actually one and the same. Thinking about wholeness in this way adds a much greater depth dimension to our connectedness. When we connect with others, with nature, and with ourselves, then we are also connecting with God. When we participate in the relational exchange, our exchange is not just with the other person, the animal, the tree, or the water, but it is also with God. This notion of continual relationality with God is the essence of living well and our path to The Living Well.

The Iron Story

In case we are a little skeptical about what happened in the cosmos nearly 14 billion years ago, there is further convincing scientific evidence for us to consider if we look at one seemingly simple element—iron. Scientists now know that elemental iron was not created on earth.[44,45] In fact, elemental iron can only be created when a red giant star converts helium into carbon and oxygen atoms which then convert to iron atoms. When most of the star's atoms change to iron, it becomes a supernova and explodes, sending iron, carbon, and oxygen into the universe. In our particular case, gravity brought iron and other elements together to form planet Earth, with iron being one of the most abundant elements in the makeup of its core.

What makes the iron story even more interesting is how iron became part of nearly everything as life evolved here on earth. All life depends on its existence. Human life requires iron, and we can obtain it from nature. Iron is found in the plants we eat, such as spinach, potatoes, peas, lentils, broccoli, wheat, raisins, and almonds. Iron is found in animals we eat, such as beef, chicken, pork, and tuna. In the human body, iron is an essential part of hemoglobin, the oxygen-carrying protein found in red blood cells. When we breathe air, the oxygen from the air goes to our lungs and binds to the hemoglobin in our blood, which then gets carried all throughout the body. If iron were not present in our red blood cells, we could not live. Life on earth has evolved because of a series of events that took place somewhere in the cosmos billions of years ago. This makes us connected to those events from our past and with nearly all that exists on earth today.

Quantum Physics

Quantum physics is the study of the smallest particles known in science—atoms and subatomic particles. Developed in the early 1900s, quantum physics has shown that the space between the matter that we can see, touch, and feel is not empty. This space is actually filled with energy, and it can be measured.[46] This type of science has shown that this energy connects all things and can even do so outside the laws of space and time. In one particular example, physicists have proven that subatomic particles appear to be entangled with each other and do so over great distances. John Bell proved the quantum entanglement theory with scientific experiments in 1964.[47] His research and others have shown that connectedness and communication take place between seemingly inert pieces of matter simultaneously and over great distances through complex fields of energy. This type of science is extraordinary and speaks volumes about connection, communication, and the relational exchange between all that exists.

Electromagnetic Fields of Energy

Scientists are just beginning to understand the electromagnetic fields of energy, sometimes called electromagnetic vibrations, that are present in nearly all things. They are certainly present and measurable among living things and appear to interact continually with the energy fields of other living things. Scientists at the Heart Math Institute in

California have been studying this phenomenon since 1991, and their research is quite compelling.[48] There is solid evidence to show that each human body has its own electromagnetic energy field that is emitted outward and affects other humans, animals, and plants.[48] Further research has shown that these energy fields are influenced by the person's emotional state, which can, in turn, influence another person's emotional state. Certainly, our human experience has always allowed us to perceive another person's emotional state by recognizing when someone is happy, sad, or angry. But we now know that a measurable vibration or energy field is emitted, and the frequency of the energy waves depends upon the person's mood. When a person is upset or anxious, the energy emitted is measured as jagged and inconsistent. But the energy wave is smooth and consistent when the mood is calm and relaxed. Interestingly, when people feel anxious and emit a jagged energy wave, they can smooth out this wave through meditation and other techniques.[48] Even more interesting is that one person's energy can influence another in either direction, jagged or smooth. This can even happen between people and their pets, and research is ongoing to show that it may also be happening between plants and humans.[48]

There are also non-bioelectromagnetic fields of energy that can be measured from non-biological matter. One such energy field is solar wind, a stream of charged energy particles that flow from the sun.[49] Additionally, the earth itself has its own geomagnetic field of energy. Both the earth and the sun have been shown to create physiological changes in the human body. Heliobiology is a branch of biology that studies how solar and geomagnetic activity affects living organisms, especially humans. A robust amount of research has shown that disruptions in energy fields have been shown to greatly influence adverse health and behavioral effects such as depression, heart attacks, melatonin/serotonin balance, and decrease the capacity to regulate thoughts, emotions, and behaviors.[50-53] Like the other scientific examples listed above, electromagnetic energy fields provide evidence that we are not separate from others or the rest of the world. We are part of a grander scheme of wholeness and are intimately interconnected.

Social Networks and Connectedness

Perhaps some of the most compelling evidence of human connectedness comes from the social science literature on social networks. Nicholas Christakis and James Fowler published a book in 2009 titled *Connected: How Your Friends' Friends' Friends Affect Everything You Feel, Think, and Do,* which outlined how connected, important, and influential we are with each other regarding our health and well-being.[54] Their research shows that we are all part of social networks of various sizes and that our networks shape us just as we also shape them. We are all important parts of a larger network, and that network of people significantly influences us. But the network as a whole is also influenced by each one of its parts too. So, the whole is important to the parts, and the parts are important to the whole.

Prior to Christakis and Flowers's work, previous research showed that each person on earth is connected by approximately six degrees of separation.[55,56] This means we could start with one person, and through their connections with others, we could connect that person to nearly every other person on the planet. This is an extraordinary story all by itself. But Christakis and Fowler take this even further to show how people are connected to one another and how influential we are to one another. Their research showed that in most cases, our attitudes, feelings, and behaviors about such things as politics, body weight, happiness, creativity, and altruism have a statistically significant influence on our social network out to three degrees of separation. This means that we can and do affect the happiness level of a friends' friends' friend to a scientifically and statistically significant degree. And we do so even if we do not know the person separated three degrees from us. For example, their research has shown that our individual happiness level has a 15% influence on our friend's happiness. But it also has a 10% influence on our friend's friend and a 6% influence on our friend's, friend's, friend.[54,57] (These percentages may not seem like much, but in 1984 a study showed that individual happiness levels increase by only 2% after being gifted $5,000.[58]) Beyond the third degree of separation, the effect loses its statistical significance. Similar statistically significant influences were shown when looking at body weight gain, political views, and with our concern for the health and well-being of others.[54,59,60] Consider this, if your social network consisted of just 20 people and those 20 people had a social network of just 20 people with no overlap, your statistically significant influence on the happiness of others extends to 8000 people! What amazing evidence of our connection with others.

The Harvard Study of Adult Development

The most robust scientific evidence to date that shows the importance of relationships comes from the Harvard Study of Adult Development.[61,62] Beginning in 1938, researchers at Harvard set out to answer the question, "What makes a good life?" Still going strong today, the study is actively collecting data on 1300 descendants of its original 724 participants. For over 80 years, the Harvard Study has tracked the same individuals, asked thousands of questions and recorded hundreds of measurements to find out what makes a life well lived. They have found that over the long course of an individual's lifetime, one crucial factor stands out as consistently and powerfully outweighing all others for its ability to help us not just to endure life but to live with high levels of physical health, mental health, and longevity. This one single important factor is good relationships.

In 2023, the current director and assistant director, Robert Waldinger and Marc Schultz, respectively, of the Harvard Study, published the comprehensive results of the study thus far. Their conclusion is this, "the single decision that can best ensure your own health and happiness…[is] to cultivate warm relationships…of all kinds."[63] Throughout the book, Waldinger and Schultz demonstrate that this is not a choice that is made only once. But rather, focusing on good relationships is an important action that is made over and over again throughout the course of a lifetime. Their results clearly show that, although not always easy, having good relationships with others can be the antidote to life's challenges and also bring great happiness, peace, and joy throughout a lifetime. This is living well![61]

COMPASSIONATE CARE CONNECTION

Considering the scientific evidence of our connection to each other and the world around us, we can begin to see overlapping patterns of information that tell an even bigger story. The singularity of our origin and its rootedness in the Divine, matched with the energy fields that flow within, between, and among all things, combined with the relationships and social flow between people, makes our relational exchanges almost tangible. Some may even go so far as to describe the energy that flows from one person to the next as love. Although scientific evidence is helpful to get us started, we don't really need it. We can already feel relationality as love in the same way we feel the love with our spouse, our pet, the ocean, and the mountains. It can hardly be explained in any other way. To love is to be relational, and to be relational is to love—which is always available in abundance. It's the "secret sauce" to health and wellness that really isn't much of a secret and likely the simple explanation for why compassionate care matters.

CHAPTER 5

WHOLENESS

"As attachment ceases to be your motivation, your actions become reflections of compassion absolute."
-Gerald May (1940-2005), American psychiatrist and theologian

Chapter One briefly discussed our American historical evolution in the late 20th Century from the Modern Era to the Postmodern Era. A few hallmark characteristics of Postmodernism include our values of cultural diversity, hybridity, and pluralism. All of these are good for our movements forward as we become more accepting of others and recognize the sameness in humanity. This can lead to a vision of wholeness where we see one fluid and interconnected universe that accepts all that is but also makes the necessary changes for the better. However, Post-Modernism also emphasizes a world of fragments due to social change and a consumeristic and capitalistic (at least in America) society that stresses individual freedom to choose one's lifestyle over that of the larger community needs. The healthcare system likewise values fragmented data that doesn't consider the whole of the patient, organization, or system. Individualism (on personal and corporate levels) seems to be driving many of the decisions and actions of our current times. These characteristics are not aligned with the true notion of wholism. On the outside, the postmodern attitude may look like an acceptance of others. Still, our continued deep entrenchments with individualism seem to drive our actions making our movements toward wholeness seem like more of a façade than a genuine vision of the whole. This seems to be true when looking at healthcare and society in general.

TRUE SELF AND SEPARATE SELF

The notion of wholeness is admittedly a difficult concept. Maybe it is better understood in ways other than using our thinking minds. The notion of wholeness is challenging because we are taught to know what we know by thinking critically, seeing the differences between this and that, and compartmentalizing. These are the skills we are taught in school and the strategies we use in our jobs for efficiency and to ensure strong outcomes, and they have certainly been effective in some ways. Unfortunately, they lead us to believe that using our minds is the only way to know. We are taught that our minds are our only tool for understanding, and we highly value our abilities to reason, think critically, and earn high marks in school. But there are more ways of knowing than just using our minds. This is one of our great challenges as we move towards wholeness—allowing our minds to be still and making room for our hearts and bodies to show us as well.

Much has been written over the past century about our personal ego. We know that it develops very early in life and helps us identify who we are and how we fit into the world. The ego helps to motivate us to achieve, discover, and move ahead. This is especially true through the first few decades of life. Our personal ego is probably a necessary part of life in many ways. But, as many have written, it is also at the core of much of our anxiety, sadness, anger, and illness.[64] The ego is always concerned with self-protection and self-preservation. Whenever we feel like we are separate from others, superior to others, or need to be in control of others or a situation, it is our ego at work. If we get offended, it is our ego. If we get defensive, it is our ego. If we are afraid, it is usually because our ego is trying to protect our self-interests. Another name for ego is the separate self. As Fr. Richard Rohr has written about on many occasions, there is more to us than our titles, accomplishments, and personal opinions about this and that.[65] There is a depth to our being that moves beyond winning the game, being right in the debate, or having a nice car and house. We are conditioned by our society to identify ourselves only with this kind of superficiality. But there is more, and the more is often referred to as our True Self. The True Self is who we are at our most fundamental and radical level. It is the shining light deep within us that is sometimes hard to see because of all the superficial stimulation of our culture.[66]

For us to move forward in the direction of wholeness, we will need to start leaving our separate selves behind and begin our journey toward discovering our True Selves. Remaining within the separate self keeps us stuck in our personal story and doesn't allow us to see the larger story—the one that recognizes that we are part of something larger, and so is everyone else. The separate self seems to be only concerned about the personal outcome or the outcomes of the groups that are important to us. On the other hand, the True Self lets go of the need for personal achievement and moves toward the collective good. The True Self experiences the world as interconnected and interdependent, where each individual is whole unto themselves but only as part of the larger wholeness of all that is.

Looking toward our True-Self is likely a new concept for us because our culture really only knows the separate self. But, for us to make any great movements toward wellness and well-being, we must, at some point in our lives, deal with the self. By that, I mean we need to come to terms with the part of ourselves that is always trying to impress, trying to be smart, trying to set ourselves apart, trying to be perfect, trying to be in control—in other words, trying to be separate and superior to feed our ego, aka our separate self. We cannot move in the direction of wellness if we do not begin to let this go. Rohr often says that this will initially feel like dying to ourselves, and most of us are afraid to go there because our ego makes us feel so good, but only superficially.[66] Discovering our True-Self is difficult because it feels like "no thing" whereas our separate self feels like something - so why would we do it? It is counter-cultural to want to move in this direction, isn't it? But we already know what it feels like to live within our True-Self if we have had just one love experience in our lives. That connection that cannot be understood with the head but rather experienced in the body and the heart, and not just the sentimental heart. It is a glimpse of our True-Self. It is what we long for in every aspect of life. It is impossible to us to live in our True-Self all the time. But the more we let down our guard and soften ourselves, the closer we get. Our current culture tells us this strategy will make us weak. But, if we do, we experience liberation and the paradox of knowing that it makes us stronger and eliminates stress along the way. So, how do we move in this direction? It starts and ends with the stillness of our thinking minds. Again, this is counter and paradoxical to what we are used to hearing. But moving forward toward wholeness is done so by doing nothing except slowing ourselves down and taking the time to sit in silence and stillness and being present to the now and being intentional about it. Moving intentionality towards nothingness is a paradoxical path toward transformation. We will discuss the action steps to move in this direction in more detail in Chapter 7.

Our ability to let go of the thinking mind's need to be in control, hold on to our titles and achievements, and see ourselves as somehow separate and more special than others is the point of the quote from Gerald May at the beginning of this chapter. A movement toward non-attachment and non-clinging is a movement toward a recognition of our True Selves. And this movement towards the True Self is a movement towards wholeness and truly living well.

TINKERING AND TRANSFORMATION

Several years ago, my colleagues and I had the opportunity to develop a brand-new major for our undergraduate students. We were challenged to design a program that offered new ways of defining health that would result in new ways of addressing health issues. In many ways, that opportunity started a new path for me, personally and professionally, and this book has become part of that journey. One of the leading programmatic outcomes that developed from that process was something we called "tinkering." We defined tinkering as the continual and reflective process of making small adjustments to health strategies that would lead to meaningful and sustainable long-term health outcomes. A few examples of these so-called tinkering strategies included enhanced physical activity, eating healthy foods, and getting quality sleep. These may seem like obvious healthy lifestyle strategies. Still, the intention and approach to their implementation are where we felt the newness in what we were developing had an opportunity to move students forward on a new path of understanding.

For several decades many have researched, written about, and presented the benefits of healthy lifestyle activities such as eating healthy, being physically active, and getting enough sleep. But our understanding of the health benefits seems to stop with our understanding of the physical benefits of these activities. We know that all three can improve health and stave off chronic illness. But, if they are done with intentionality and relationality, they may also move us toward transformation and a depth dimension that leads to wholeness and a truer sense of living well.

Tinkering is the action necessary on our end by putting us in a position to be aware of the relational exchange that is always present. It is the very participation and intention that is so important and necessary to our movement toward wholeness. But tinkering is not the end of the journey. It is a conduit for the path toward transformation. Most wellness programs focus on tinkering only without the purposeful connection to transformation—what we might call disconnected tinkering. We are moving in the right direction but not going far enough to make the connection. Tinkering can put us in a position to move toward transformation if we allow it to do so. This is a key to transformation and wholeness. Our True Self is already and always present as a gift. It is who God is and whom God knows us to be. Unfortunately, we often get stuck in our separate ego-driven selves. We cannot see and recognize that our True Self is present under all the layers of the perceptions of our social and cultural expectations and pressures. But, if we intentionally put ourselves in a position to receive, we can recognize the wholeness within ourselves and others, which is a movement towards transformation and wholeness.

ONEING AND WONING

Our ability to move towards transformation means we are not a fixed entity. We are not stuck where we are. We can move and evolve into something different, more, and with greater depth. This includes the relational exchange and the non-clinging to our separate self-idealism discussed above, and it is a movement towards a unitive existence of higher consciousness. One of the hallmarks of our separate self way of seeing is our dualistic view of the world. This way of seeing recognizes only the differences that exist between people. If you are of one political position, you likely think the other side is wrong, and you are right. If you are of one religious faith, you likely think yours is right and others are wrong. This binary way of thinking may be the same for your gender preference, race preference, and your favorite sports team. Dualistic thinking is a "won-ing" type of thinking where if I am for "this," then I must be against "that." It is competition driven and leads to disconnection rather than connection and unity. Living with a woning attitude is living with an attitude of being separate from other people except for those like me and/or my groups.

The alternate way of living is one of non-dualism or unitive existence. This way of seeing the world was described so beautifully by the English mystic Julian of Norwich (1343-after 1416) as "Oneing"—and is the opposite of woning.[67] As a noun, Oneing is union. And, as a verb, Oneing is the connectedness action that brings all things together. Seeing the connectedness, sameness, and singleness of all that is, is Oneing. That is to say, the unified wholeness of everything where we no longer focus on the characteristics that separate and make us different (man v woman, black v white, old v young). We only see the world through "singleness" – or unified consciousness. Once we begin to see in this way, we become less critical and nihilistic, and we soften to accept "what is." It's also important to understand that this way of seeing doesn't mean we stand still and let the world play out without our input. It's just the opposite. We engage where and when needed and to the degree necessary to make life better for those in need.

WHOLENESS IN HEALTHCARE

As stated earlier, the concepts of wholeness can be challenging to understand. Many of the terms used to describe wholeness, such as non-dualism, singleness, and Oneing have overlapping meanings, and all point in the same direction. Non-dualism is becoming more consciously aware of living in the now and in unity with all that is. Singleness is the ability to see the interchangeability and fluidity of all that is. It is also a recognition of no beginning, no end, no good, and no evil. There is just an is-ness to everything without labels. These are challenging concepts, to be sure. But if we can hold the tension we feel in our minds as we struggle with what we thought were opposites and accept them as part of our being, as being part of the whole, then we can also start to let go of many other labels as well. If we can begin to recognize that all that exists, including our attitudes and opinions, is part of a grand and interconnected whole, we can also recognize that what we thought were opposites (conservatives and liberals, Pro-Life and Pro-Choice, joy and suffering, life and death) are not opposites at all but rather all important parts of the same wholeness. This way of seeing allows space in our minds and hearts for everything and softens us to what and who we thought were our enemies, and creates a more unified existence. It creates Oneing and moves us toward the meaning of living well and most assuredly leads us to The Living Well.

Within the context of healthcare professionals and the systems within which we work, seeing through the lens of Oneing can change our perspectives. Rather than blaming the system for its inefficiencies and lack of regard for the personnel working to make it better, we can see ourselves and the system as co-creators of something better. The conversations change from us versus them to a unitive and collective responsibility. The blame is no longer on something out there because the something out there includes me too. And this Oneing perspective is not just from the perspective of the individual—it includes the system seeing itself as part of the greater whole as well. Oneing allows everyone to see and accept the is-ness of the current situation while at the same time more clearly seeing what is necessary to make improvements. This is a collective and unified movement towards living well for everyone.

CHAPTER 6

TOWARDS

"Personal participation is the universal principle of knowing."
-Michael Polanyi (1891-1976), British Scientist and Philosopher

In the previous chapter, we discussed both the True Self and the separate self and the notion that the True Self is already present. Which is to say, we are already whole. If this is true, then it naturally begs the question, "If I am already whole, why do I need to do anything to experience this wholeness?" This is one of the great mysteries of life. But, as many have said, God is both hidden and everywhere at the same time, and God loves to be known.[68,69] In other words, some action is required from us to know God more fully. Polanyi's message above is fitting—our personal [and collective] participation in the exchange is a necessary requirement for our movement toward wholeness.

INTENTIONALITY

Intentionality is our authentic and conscious desire to do something. It is our purposeful "Yes" to be part of something. A movement towards wholeness doesn't seem to be possible on its own. We must agree in some way to be part of it through a conscious and authentic desire. This is our action to move forward.

In our customary way of life, our lifeworld, we tend to solve all problems with actions. Most often, we feel like it is our responsibility to make everything correct through an action of some kind. Sometimes this is called the "righting reflex." But the action we are talking about through intentionality is different and more subtle than our default urge to fix. Yes, it is an action. But most often, it doesn't look like the items on our traditional "to-do" lists or the "can-do" attitude that our forefathers used to tame the West in America. Thinking back to our discussions in the previous chapter about the True Self, our righting reflex may look at it and say we are already there. There is nothing left to do. But we must resist the notion that because our True Self and wholeness are already present, inaction is our way forward. We are co-creators with God in our evolution; therefore, we must engage and do something. But, from the outsider's view, this "something" may seem like nothing. In the previous chapter, we discussed the seemingly "nothingness" of stillness required of us to move toward transformation and wholeness. Our intentional "Yes" to the stillness is, in fact, an action. When we desire to move toward wholeness, this is intentionality. This is our "Yes" and our agreement to be part of the evolutionary process with God. Our action is to simply participate with an authentic and conscious "Yes!"

DISCOVERING WHAT IS OURS TO DO

Intentionality is a good place to begin our conversation about our movement toward wholeness, but it doesn't seem to provide a great deal of clarity about what we are actually to do. Having the desire to move towards wholeness puts us in a position, so to speak. We are in the right posture with our intentional participation. But what is it that we are to do? What is our purpose, our calling, our vocation? These questions help move us closer to wholeness and to living well, especially as healthcare professionals working in a challenging environment.

Much has been written about discovering our purpose. Scientific literature shows us that being able to discern and write our life purpose can lead to all kinds of health benefits.[70] Just being conscious of our purpose has been shown to promote healthy aging, enhance sleep quality, encourage healthier eating habits, increase energy, reduce stroke and heart attack risk, lower the stress hormone cortisol, improve the management of diabetes, and lower depression.[70] Knowing our purpose is clearly important to living well. But it is also important to understand that our purpose should not be limited to having more money, fame, status, higher academic degrees, better grades, etc. Our life purpose and the health benefits that can be achieved have a greater depth dimension than surface-level accomplishments.

Nearly everything written about the topic of purpose is about what we believe we are to do in this world. In other words, what actions are we to take, and what tasks are we to perform during our lifetime? For example, my purpose within my work life is to lead students toward wholeness. In my home life, my purpose is to be the best husband and father I can be. And in my personal life, my purpose is to serve as an example of kindness to all. [*my actual life purpose statements*] Certainly, these are good and even necessary. They point me in a direction at work, at home, and within my personal life. But I have discovered that they may not be going far enough. They may be stuck in our American action-oriented way of life.

Eckhart Tolle has done some writing in the area of purpose and has some interesting insights that can lead us toward a greater depth dimension. As he says, our lives have both an outer and inner purpose.[71] We tend only to consider our outer action-oriented purpose. This is because so much of our lives are focused on achievement. But our inner purpose is separate. Our inner purpose concerns our "being" and is our primary purpose. Our outer purpose concerns our "doing" and is secondary. But they are both good and necessary. Therefore, aligning our inner and outer purpose is important as a posturing movement toward wholeness. Our inner being and inner purpose is our True Self, and when we give an intentional "Yes" to this purpose, we can also be more intentional with our outer purpose. This can set a pathway of relationality to the whole, as discussed in Chapter Four.

The Center for Action and Contemplation has provided a great deal of clarity on the confusion around "How do I know what is mine to do?".[72] This was a topic from their Daily Meditation in August of 2022.[72] Within the reflection, Fr. Richard and the CAC staff explain that everything can be seen as guidance from a greater Source. The reflection says, "Our ability to trust that there is guidance available allows it to *become* guidance! Basically, we switch from the fixing, fully understanding, and controlling mode to the trusting, listening, and allowing mode. Then we start allowing the Divine Flow instead of stopping it with a "no" or a question mark."[72] Fr. Richard Rohr takes this notion further as he explains that the "knowing" actually comes from the stillness…"From my own experience, I know I need a contemplative practice. Some form of the prayer of quiet is necessary to touch me at the unconscious level, the level where deep and lasting transformation occurs. From my place of prayer, I am able to understand more clearly what is mine to do and have the courage to do it."[72] Contemplation allows us to set aside the dualistic notion that our actions are about competition and winning. We no longer need this as our motivation. We only need to do what we have to do. Our contemplative interior work leads to the clarity we need for our active exterior work that is uniquely ours to do, but at the same time, work that is deeply connected with all others. For some, this is activism, but for others, it is teaching. For some, it is public-level care, but for others, it is care at the individual level. We should be careful not to be tempted by the guilt of needing to solve all the world's problems just by our actions alone. Our work together is complex and highly connected; we just need to do what is ours to do while allowing others to do the same. This can also be said at the institutional and corporate levels in healthcare. Do what is ours to do at the institutional levels through our collective contemplation.

Intentionality is a movement. It is a movement not to perfect but rather to move in the direction of, which is to say, the direction of transformation and wholeness. Intentionality is both action and contemplation at the same time. It is striving and moving toward something new at the same time as accepting what is now. Holding these concepts together both individually and collectively is a movement toward living well as healthcare professionals within the healthcare system.

CHAPTER 7

POSTURING

"To be still, yet still moving, that is everything."
-Do Hyun Choe

If we were to go to the dictionary and look up the word posture, we would find several definitions. As a noun, the standard definition of posture means the position in which we hold our bodies. But also, as a noun, it means a particular way of dealing with or considering something.[73] Additionally, as a verb, posture means to place oneself in a particular attitude or pose. When I began writing this book, the meaning I was using for posture was the latter—to place oneself in a certain kind of attitude and, in particular, an attitude that is open to receiving a relational exchange with all that exists. However, now that we are toward the end of the book, I think the meaning of posture as a noun works, too. There is a way of knowing that takes place through our bodies as much as through our minds, and our posture has a lot to do with that, both literally and figuratively. And the second definition of posture as a noun may be the best of all. The notion of wholeness and moving towards it as a way of living well is, at minimum, something to consider, as the definition states. Posturing is both an action and an attitude. It is a way to consider putting ourselves in a position to receive as well as a position to give. To consider posturing is to consider the relational exchange that moves us towards wholeness and living well as healthcare professionals.

We have spent the previous six chapters diving into challenging concepts that move us toward transformation and wholeness. But, ironically, the "how to" is quite simple. This isn't to say that posturing is easy. In fact, for most of us, it seems quite difficult because it goes against our cultural standard norms. Most often, posturing looks like nothing. There is no objective to achieve anything or do anything and there are no goals associated with the action of posturing. It is more about our participation in posturing than it is about our perfection and achievement. Only presence is required. Our action-focused and achievement-obsessed minds will likely have difficulty with the stillness that is necessary for posturing toward wholeness. But, if we are patient, we can experience a sense of peace and happiness (not to mention less stress and burnout) that goes far beyond all the action-oriented strategies combined that we have tried in the past.

CONTEMPLATION IN PRACTICE

Etymologically, contemplation comes from the Latin word *contemplatio*, meaning "to gaze attentively." Some have described contemplation as the act of bringing forward a new consciousness that is needed to awaken a more loving, just, and sustainable world.[74] Others have simply described it as taking a long and loving look.[64] Contemplation involves seeing, hearing, and feeling, but with more than our eyes, ears, and fingertips. Contemplation involves being fully present in our hearts, minds, and bodies at the same time. It transcends us to a way of knowing that goes beyond our thinking minds and our sentimental hearts. It enables us to know more deeply and allows us to respond creatively and work toward what could be.[74] Contemplation brings about consciousness that leads to a clarity of action and a knowing of what is ours to do.

Healthcare, not unlike many other institutions, is a large system rooted in capitalistic idealism while also trying to balance the morality of caring for each other. The tension that exists in trying to maintain a balance between the two has led us to the fatigue, burnout, and chronic stress that was the impetus of this book. Adopting a more contemplative stance may help to gently mitigate the widespread stress being placed on providers, patients, and the system itself. And the kind of contemplation we are speaking of here is not just at the level of the individual person. If embraced at the group, organizational, corporate, and system levels, the structural factors that lead to personal strain can be mitigated too. For an organization to move to a level of knowing that provides clarity about what is theirs to do [as an interconnected organization] could provide more compassion and stress relief to the people inside the organization. At the same time, if the individuals within the organization are also becoming more conscious about what is theirs to do [as interconnected individuals] through contemplative practices, they could provide relief to their own personal stress, that of their patients and coworkers, and also that of the organization. This is seeing through the whole that cannot be done just with the eyes. This is an act of Oneing and non-dualism where everyone within the organization is able to see that they are whole, but only because they are part of the larger whole.

St. Ignatius of Loyola is credited for teaching others to be contemplatives in action. He knew that when we move to a deeper level of consciousness we can see, hear, and feel differently than before. And it is this greater awareness and knowing that then guides our actions. Healthcare can do the same. If the structural system of a healthcare organization and the people within the organization move toward this deeper level of consciousness together, all the parts will co-creatively move [posture] toward wholeness. It could then be said that the whole organization is contemplative in the practice of healthcare and could provide great relief to the tensions that currently exist.

POSTURING PRACTICE

Putting ourselves in a position of relational exchange is admittedly confusing. However, it really only requires two things from us. The first is intentionality, an authentic and genuine intention to be open to the present as it is, and the second is patience. The first is our "Yes" to move in this direction with faith, vulnerability, trust, and courage. This is our "action" part of the relational exchange, which looks like stillness (as we will see below). The second, our patience, may be even more difficult than the first. It is the receiving part of the exchange. It is difficult because it is pure Grace and Love. The receiving comes in its own time, and what comes is always enough.

There are three contemplative practices that are outlined in this chapter. However, there are an endless number of ways to practice contemplation. When we are more present in the now, we are more aware, more conscious, and more open. We are able to see, hear, and feel with more of ourselves, and this is contemplation. It can take place anywhere and at any time without the need to set aside more time in our day and make room for something else to do. It is always accessible and is always enough. But, for most of us, creating the kind of stillness that is required for contemplation in the middle of a busy day is difficult for our overstimulated and overworked minds and bodies. Therefore, certain exercises are helpful that can make room for stillness.

The three exercises below were chosen because they each approach contemplation from a different starting point. The Ignatian Daily Examen initially uses the mind and the practice of reflection as the starting point. Centering Prayer uses the heart as its starting point and the Welcoming Prayer uses the body. As we have mentioned several times throughout this book, there are more ways of knowing than just through our thinking minds. We seem to be most familiar with using this method to know what we know because it has been our culturally approved default system. However, using our hearts and our bodies is equally as important. As we move to greater levels of consciousness, we use all three at the same time to know what we know rather than compartmentalizing them into just one. Although each of the three practices of contemplation shown below begins within its own space, each widens to include the other ways of knowing with time. It may be a good idea to start with one practice that seems to be the best fit at the moment and then move to the others when the timing is right. In other words, if you best resonate with mind-centered reflective activities, start with the Ignatian Daily Examen. Practice contemplation in this way and then move on to another practice when you are ready to try a different starting point. It doesn't matter where you start, just that you have a genuine desire for a relational exchange.

The Ignatian Daily Examen

The Examen is an ancient practice of prayerful reflection that has been used in the Catholic Church as a way to recognize God's relational exchange with us as we move about our day. It is a technique of prayerful reflection to help us see, hear, and feel God's presence in all people, all things, and all the happenings of life. It helps us to recognize God in all our experiences. There are many versions of the Examen, but the one presented here is a technique that

St. Ignatius of Loyola used within his Spiritual Exercises and that which he taught others. He required his Jesuit priests to practice The Examen twice daily and many still recommend practicing this exercise one to two times daily for about twenty minutes. The following five steps are those that Ignatius taught his followers:

1. Move to a quiet place, take a couple of deep breaths, and become aware that God is present just as you are.
2. Reflect on the events of the day in your mind, those that were easy to receive and those that were difficult to receive, with gratitude.
3. Pay particular attention to the emotions you feel from these events.
4. Choose one feature from the day that continues to draw your attention and remain with that feature in stillness.
5. Ask God to keep you open to the events of tomorrow.

The Examen asks us to reflect on the events of the day and to receive them as they are, not judging whether they are good or bad but simply allowing them to be. If there is one event that produces a particularly strong feeling, stay with that experience and try to recognize the gifts that it brings. For more information and details about each step of the Ignatian Daily Examen, visit Ignatian Spirituality and their website at: https://www.ignatianspirituality.com.

The Centering Prayer

Centering Prayer, developed by Fr. Thomas Keating and his colleagues, is a contemplative prayer designed to help our whole selves receive the gift of greater consciousness through our hearts. Fr. Keating described Centering Prayer as a relationship with God and a practice to help foster that relationship. The practice of Centering Prayer is a receptive method of silent prayer that moves us beyond a conversation with God and into communion with God.[75,76] There are four simple steps to Centering Prayer that can be practiced one to two times daily. It is recommended to begin with as little as five minutes and move toward twenty minutes. The steps include:

1. Choose a sacred word as a symbol of your intention to consent to God's presence and action within.

2. Sitting comfortably and with your eyes closed, settle briefly and silently and introduce the sacred word as a symbol of your consent and action to God's presence within.
3. When engaged with your thoughts, return ever-so-gently to your sacred word.
4. At the end of the prayer period, remain in silence with eyes closed for a couple of minutes.

The steps of the Centering Prayer are brief and simple, but this exercise can be difficult. As you may have noticed, there is nothing to do after introducing your sacred word but to remain open to God. There is nothing to think about and no words to recite. Just stillness. And that is the main point of the exercise—to not focus your attention on anything. It is natural and normal for thoughts to enter the mind, mostly because our lives are so filled with stimulation and our minds want to work and do something constantly. But this exercise is exactly the opposite. The Centering Prayer is only stillness and openness to God that already dwells within. And when our minds wander towards thoughts or our attention has moved to a sound or feeling, we ever-so-gently let it go and return to our sacred word and the stillness of our being. The point of Centering Prayer is not to see how long we can be still but rather the letting go and return to the stillness. This may happen hundreds of times throughout a prayer session, and that is okay. It's the letting go that is important, not the holding on, which is the key to this contemplative prayer. For more information on the Centering Prayer, please visit the Contemplative Outreach at https://www.contemplativeoutreach.org/centering-prayer-method/.

The Welcoming Prayer

The Welcoming Prayer uses the body as the entry point into contemplation. It is a method of consenting to God's presence and action in our physical selves. For example, within our situational daily lives, we frequently experience emotions that are sometimes difficult to receive. We experience sadness, frustration, anger, and sometimes pain. But we also experience joy, happiness, exhilaration, and pleasure. The purpose of the Welcoming Prayer is to deepen our relationship with God by consenting to these bodily feelings as they

are happening. It is easy to accept and consent to the feelings we label as good. But what about those that are more difficult to receive, like pain and sadness? As explained by the Contemplative Outreach Center, "Welcoming Prayer helps us to dismantle our acquired emotional programs and to heal the wounds of a lifetime where they are stored – in the body."
[https://www.contemplativeoutreach.org/welcoming-prayer-method/]

There are just three steps to the Welcoming Prayer:

1. Feel and sink into what you are experiencing in your body at this moment.
2. Welcome what you are experiencing at this moment in your body as an opportunity to consent to the Divine Indwelling. Some recommend naming what you are feeling.
3. Let go by saying silently, "I let go of my desire for security, affection, and control, and embrace this moment as it is."

It is recommended that we start with the little things of everyday life that cause frustration, like sitting in traffic or waiting in line at the grocery store. The initial step is to recognize what we are feeling, followed by our genuine intention of welcoming the feeling. We can even name the feeling if we want. After some time, we allow ourselves to let the feeling go. Just as we did to our thoughts in the Centering Prayer, we ever-so-gently let go. The continual act of letting go, sometimes called kenosis, then becomes an action pattern with more practice. The letting go process then becomes part of our relational exchange. A bit of caution here, though—try not to be confused that kenosis means apathy and that we shouldn't work to make changes to bad situations. These contemplative exercises provide a greater consciousness and clarity that helps us to know what is ours to do when changes are needed.

As we become more comfortable with using the Welcoming Prayer for small situations, we can move toward larger situations that have more deeply seeded feelings that we store in the body. The process of letting go eventually leads to freedom and liberation by ridding ourselves of that which binds us and holds us back from a life well lived.

As mentioned above, the three contemplative exercises described in this chapter are just the tip of the iceberg. The opportunities for experiencing increased awareness of the present through greater levels of consciousness are everywhere. Greater consciousness can be experienced when we are with other people. Greater consciousness can be experienced while we exercise, after getting a good night's sleep, or by improving our eating habits. Greater consciousness can be experienced through our relational exchange with nature as we listen to the birds sing or feel the breeze on our face and see it rustle the leaves of a tree. Greater consciousness can be experienced while drawing, painting, singing, and dancing. And greater consciousness can be experienced through many forms of meditation, prayer, and religious services from many types of religions. The list is endless because God is present in everyone and everything—including ourselves. Consenting to the relational exchange of a certain moment within our busy day means we become aware that we receive something from someone or something else, and in return, we give something of ourselves as if it were a dance. It would be impossible (and probably impractical) to remain in a contemplative posture at every moment of every day. But pausing our lives for even a moment to recognize the connection allows us to move toward wholeness.

POSTURING AS A HEALTHCARE PROFESSIONAL

Becoming a contemplative in practice may initially seem like a stretch for some who practice in the complex, overworked, and overburdened healthcare system. But we already know that making a connection with patients makes a difference in their lives—and ours. We know that working within a positive environment of an organization that cares for our personal well-being matters. Within those relationships are relational exchanges that don't just feed our minds but our hearts and bodies too. Becoming more contemplative so that we can be more conscious gives us what we need to do what is ours to do, and to know what we should leave for others to do. The stillness that is needed in contemplation guides our actions. The quote at the beginning of this chapter from Do Hyun Choe says, "to be still, yet still moving, that is everything," could not be better stated. Being a contemplative in practice is a movement toward wholeness. When we regularly put ourselves in a position to receive from others and to give of ourselves to others, it guides our actions both personally and professionally. The abundance of the intentional dance of the relational exchange places us in a position to be more contemplative, more conscious, and more compassionate. This is the dance toward wholeness and our radical way forward to living well as healthcare professionals.

EMERGING THOUGHTS

As we come to a close, I cannot help but think there is much more work to do in this space. It hardly seems fitting to even name these final thoughts as conclusions because it feels more like a beginning. Yet, everything presented throughout this book has already been said before. Philosophers, psychologists, sociologists, mystics, and spiritual teachers have been writing about the deeper importance of connection and relationship for (literally) thousands of years. So, it seems strange that anyone should feel moved to write yet another book about the topic, especially a book for those whose job it is to care for others. The topics discussed throughout this book were directed towards healthcare professionals, but hopefully, you are able to see they are universal to life itself, regardless of occupation. But specific to those who work in healthcare, the very nature of the job is built upon connection and relationship. Most people feel called to work in healthcare because they have the desire to help others. But somehow, we got a bit sidetracked and distracted by culturally accepted norms (lifeworlds) that turned this desire (at least on a system level, anyway) into a primary focus on standardized metrics, electronic medical records, and the economic bottom line. Our longing to be connected to others and to have an influence on relieving human suffering has been superseded with numbers and outcomes, leaving those who are charged with alleviating the suffering of others with their own kind of suffering. Despite our tendencies for individualism, the human experience longs for connection. And not just a connection with each other, but with nature, with ourselves, and with God. Unfortunately, living in our Modern/Post-Modern world and working within a system such as healthcare doesn't seem to allow for the capacity to meet our most fundamental needs for connection. At times, the impossibility of the context just seems too great.

The purpose of this book was to take a deeper dive into our understanding of this fundamental need for connection and relationship so that we can better understand what it means to live well. The overarching message is rather simple—if we can put ourselves in a position (both literally and figuratively) to be aware of and participate in a relational exchange with others, nature, God, and even ourselves, then we may be able to move toward this radical and fundamental part of ourselves that is already present and whole in spite of a system that doesn't seem to support or value this need. In other words, our enhanced awareness and participation in relationality allows us to get to a greater depth dimension of our lives that moves beyond the superficiality of our lifeworlds and centers us closer to a wholeness and True Self that already exists regardless of occupation or its structural limitations. This movement doesn't mean we leave behind the world as we know it. It actually brings us closer to it by having a foot in both camps at the same time. This movement towards wholeness allows us to accept the world as it is and, at the same time, work to make the injustices better—and not just within the healthcare system but in all aspects of life.

So much evidence points to our continued struggles with stress, fatigue, and burnout that it is easy for some to believe that living well may not be a reality for those working in healthcare. Much has been written about what can be done to improve this public health crisis and it is my hope that research in this area will continue to evolve in the coming months and years. What I also hope has become clear after reading this book, however, is that the radical solutions that are needed are not so radical after all. At the most fundamental (and radical) level, relationships appear to be the heart of the issue. We have more than enough scientific proof to show that compassion for others offers a relational exchange that benefits both the receiver and the giver. And we have seen that the importance of these relationships is not just limited to the patient and the provider. Relational exchanges are the heart of living well when they include co-workers, leadership, and the organization and system, too. But they don't stop there. Being conscious of the continual giving and receiving (the Dance) that happens with all that is allows us to recognize that we are part of something much larger than ourselves and that these relationships are critical for us to live well.

We began this book journey in the *Preface* with the quote, "How you do anything is how you do everything." Our ever-expanding and evolving consciousness toward wholeness allows us to know that we are whole unto ourselves, but only when we realize that we are part of the larger whole. Right intentionality within our actions is not just right here and now but right everywhere. If we can be conscious of the flow (which is to say, the love) that we exchange within our relationships, we are evolving toward wholeness and living well. The "posturing" action presented in this book is not based on achieving or attaining anything because nothing is missing. The wholeness that we seek is already present. Therefore, the real action that is necessary is to let go of what hinders us from realizing it.

REFERENCES

1. Freudenberger HJ. Staff Burn-Out. *Journal of Social Issues*. 1974;30:159-165. https://doi.org/10.1111/j.1540-4560.1974.tb00706.x

2. Maslach C, Jackson SE. The Measurement of Experienced Burnout. *J Organiz Behav*. 1981;2:99-113. https://doi.org/10.1002/job.4030020205

3. American Medical Association. Physician Burnout Rate Spikes to New Height. September 15, 2022. Available at: https://www.ama-assn.org/press-center/press-releases/physician-burnout-rate-spikes-new-height. Accessed on March 17, 2023.

4. Sulmaz G, Bagheri LK, Mohammad Y, Keyvan H, Saeed S, Sajjad A. A systematic review and meta-analysis of burnout among healthcare workers during COVID-19. *Frontiers in Psychiatry*. 2021;12. https://www.frontiersin.org/articles/10.3389/fpsyt.2021.758849

5. United States Census Bureau. 22 million employed in health care fight against COVID-19. April 5, 2021. Available at: https://www.census.gov/library/stories/2021/04/who-are-our-health-care-workers.html. Accessed on: March 17, 2023.

6. Tawfik DS, Profit J, Morgenthaler TI, et al. Physician burnout, well-being, and work unit safety grades in relationship to reported medical errors. *Mayo Clinic Proceedings*. 2018;93(11):1571-1580.

7. Andel C, Davidow SL, Hollander M, Moreno DA. The economics of healthcare quality and medical errors. *Journal of Health Care Finance*. 2012;39(1):39-50.

8. Peckham C. Medscape national physician burnout & depression report. Medscape. 2018.

9. Young A, Chaudhry HJ, Pei X, Arnhart K, Dugan M, Snyder GB. A census of actively licensed physicians in the United States, 2016. *Journal of Medical Regulation*. 2017;103(2):7-21.

10. American Medical Association. Creating the organizational foundation for joy in medicine. Available at: https://edhub.ama-assn.org/steps-forward/module/2702510. Accessed on March 17, 2023.

11. Anderson P. Physicians experience highest suicide rate of any profession. Medscape Medical News. Published electronically May 7, 2018.

12. Dyrbye LN, Shanafelt TD, Sinsky CA, et al. Burnout among healthcare professionals: A call to explore and address this underground threat to safe, high-quality care. *NAM Perspectives*. Discussion Paper, National Academy of Medicine, Washington, DC. 2017. https://doi.org/10.31478/201707b

13. Trzeciak S, Mazzarelli A. *Compassionomics: The revolutionary scientific evidence that caring makes a difference*. Chicago, IL: Huron Consulting Group, 2019.

14. Burton R. *The Anatomy of Melancholy*. London, UK: 1621

15. American Psychological Association. Stress in America 2022. October 2022. Available at: https://www.apa.org/news/press/releases/stress/2022/concerned-future-inflation. Accessed on March 17, 2023.

16. American Institute of Stress. What is stress? Available at: https://www.stress.org/daily-life. Accessed on March 17, 2023.

17. National Institute for Occupational Safety and Health. Centers for Disease Control and Prevention. Health Worker Mental Health. May 11, 2022. Available at: https://www.cdc.gov/niosh/newsroom/feature/health-worker-mental-health.html. Accessed on March 17, 2023.

18. National Institute for Occupational Safety and Health. Centers for Disease Control and Prevention. Health Worker Mental Health. Work and fatigue. March 2, 2023. Available at: https://www.cdc.gov/niosh/topics/fatigue/default.html#:~:text=Fatigue%20has%20been%20described%20as,work%20and%20extended%20work%20hours. Accessed on March 17, 2023.

19. Sadeghniiat-Haghighi K, Yazdi Z. Fatigue management in the workplace. *Ind Psychiatry J*. 2015 Jan-Jun;24(1):12-7. doi: 10.4103/0972-6748.160915. PMID: 26257477; PMCID: PMC4525425.

20. American Psychological Association. APA Dictionary of Psychology. Burnout. Available at: https://dictionary.apa.org/burnout. Accessed on March 17, 2023.

21. Brindley PG, Olusanya S, Wong A, Crowe L, Hawryluck L. Psychological 'burnout' in healthcare professionals: Updating our understanding, and not making it worse. *Journal of the Intensive Care Society.* 2019;20(4):358–362.

22. Seaward BL. *Managing Stress. Principles and Strategies for Health and Well-Being,* 7th Ed. Jones & Bartlett Learning. Burlington, MA. 2012.

23. American Institute of Stress. Stress Research. 2014 Stress Statistics. http://www.stress.org. Accessed on December 2, 2019.

24. Miller GE, Chen E, Zhou ES. If it goes up, must it come down? Chronic stress and the hypothalamic-pituitary-adrenocortical axis in humans. *Psychological Bulletin*. 2007;133(1):25-45.

25. American Psychological Association. Stress in America 2021. October 26, 2021. Available at: https://www.apa.org/news/press/releases/stress/2021/october-decision-making. Accessed on March 18, 2023.

26. Palsson OS, Ballou S, Gray S. The U.S. National Pandemic Emotional Impact Report. June 2020. Available at: Available at: https://pandemicimpactreport.com/. Accessed on March 18, 2023.

27. American Psychological Association. APA's 2021 Work and Well-Being Survey results. The American workforce faces compounding pressure. Available at: https://www.apa.org/pubs/reports/work-well-being/compounding-pressure-2021. Accessed on March 18, 2023.

28. Russell, G., Lightman, S. The human stress response. *Nat Rev Endocrinol* **15**, 525–534 (2019). https://doi.org/10.1038/s41574-019-0228-0

29. Harvard Medical School. Special Health Report: *Stress Management: Enhance your well-being by reducing stress and building resilience*. Harvard Health Publications. Harvard University. Boston. 2016.

30. McFarland MJ, Hayward MD. Poverty and Awakening Cortisol in Adolescence: The Importance of Timing in Early Life. *Soc Ment Health*. 2014 Mar;4(1):21-37. doi: 10.1177/2156869313500278. PMID: 26140229; PMCID: PMC4485454.

31. McFarland MJ, Hayward MD. Poverty and Awakening Cortisol in Adolescence: The Importance of Timing in Early Life. *Soc Ment Health*. 2014 Mar;4(1):21-37. doi: 10.1177/2156869313500278. PMID: 26140229; PMCID: PMC4485454.

32. Townsend SS, Major B, Gangi CE, Mendes WB. From "in the air" to "under the skin": cortisol responses to social identity threat. *Pers Soc Psychol Bull*. 2011 Feb;37(2):151-64. doi: 10.1177/0146167210392384. PMID: 21239591; PMCID: PMC3538844.

33. Scandurra C, Carbone A, Baiocco R, Mezzalira S, Maldonato NM, Bochicchio V. Gender Identity Milestones, Minority Stress and Mental Health in Three Generational Cohorts of Italian Binary and Nonbinary Transgender People. *International Journal of Environmental Research and Public Health*. 2021; 18(17):9057. https://doi.org/10.3390/ijerph18179057.

34. Yao B, Meng L, Hao M, Zhang Y, Gong T, Guo Z. Chronic stress: A critical risk factor for atherosclerosis. *Journal of International Medical Research* 2019, Vol. 47(4) 1429–1440.

35. Murthy V. Addressing health worker burnout. The U.S. Surgeon General's Advisory on Building a Thriving Health Workforce. Office of the U.S. Surgeon General. United States Department of Health and Human Services. Available at:

https://www.hhs.gov/surgeongeneral/priorities/health-worker-burnout/index.html. Accessed on: March 18, 2023.

36. Teilhard de Chardin P. *The Phenomenon of Man.* (English translation by Bernard Wall) William Collins Sons and Co. London. 1959.

37. Seligman ME. *Flourish: A visionary new understanding of happiness and well-being.* Free Press, Simon & Schuster. New York. 2011.

38. Hannigan B, Edwards D, Burnard P. Stress and stress management in clinical psychology: Findings from a systematic review, *Journal of Mental Health.* 2004;13(3):235-245, DOI: 10.1080/09638230410001700871

39. Lenz TL. Chronically American: Our evolution towards chronic illness and our radical way forward. Omaha, NE: Independent Publisher, 2020.

40. Forghani N, Keshtiaray N, Yousefy A. A critical examination of postmodernism based on religious and moral value education. *International Education Studies.* 2015;8(9):98-106.

41. Habermas J. *The Theory of Communicative Action, Volume Two. Lifeworld and System: A Critique of Functionalist Reason.* (translated by McCarthy T). Beacon Press. Boston. 1987.

42. McIntosh D. Language, Self, and Lifeworld in Habermas's "Theory of Communicative Action". *Theory and Society.* 1994;23(1):1-33.

43. Turner MS. Origins of the universe. *Scientific American.* SA Special Editions. 2013;22(2s):36-43.

44. Sheftel AD, Mason AB, Ponka P. The long history of iron in the Universe and in health and disease. *Biochim Biophys Acta.* 2012 Mar;1820(3):161-87. doi: 10.1016/j.bbagen.2011.08.002. Epub 2011 Aug 9. PMID: 21856378; PMCID: PMC3258305.

45. American Museum of Natural History. We are stardust. Available at: https://www.amnh.org/exhibitions/permanent/the-universe/stars/a-spectacular-stellar-finale/we-are-stardust. Accessed on March 18, 2023.

46. Wheeler JA, Zurek WH, (eds). *Quantum Theory and Measurements.* Princeton University Press. Princeton, NJ. 1983.

47. Delio I. *A Hunger for Wholeness: Soul, Space, and Transcendence.* Paulist Press. New York. 2018.

48. McCraty R. *Science of the Heart: Exploring the role of the heart in human performance.* HeartMath Institute. Boulder Creek, CA. 2015.

49. McCraty R, Deyhle A. *The Science of Interconnectivity*. HeartMath Institute. Boulder Creek, CA. 2016.

50. Kay RW. Geomagnetic storms: Association with incidence of depression as measured by hospital admission. *British Journal of Psychiatry*. 1994;164:403-409.

51. Malin SRC. Correlation between heart attacks and magnetic activity. *Nature*. 1979;277:646-648.

52. Burch JB, Reif JS, Yost MG. Geomagnetic disturbances are associated with reduced nocturnal excretion of a melatonin metabolite in humans. *Neuroscience Letters*. 1999;266:209-212.

53. McCraty R, Shaffer F. Heart rate variability: New perspectives of physiological mechanisms, assessment of self-regulatory capacity, and health risk. *Global Advances in Health and Medicine*. 2015;4:46-61.

54. Christakis NA, Fowler JH. *Connected: How your friends' friends' friends affect everything you feel, think, and do.* Little Brown and Company. New York. 2009.

55. Travers J, Milgram S. An experimental study in the small world problem. *Sociometry*. 1969;35(4):425-443.

56. Dodds PS, et al. An experimental study of search in global social networks. *Science*. 2003;301:827-829.

57. Fowler JH, Christakis NA. Dynamic spread of happiness in a large social network: Longitudinal analysis over 20 years in the Framingham Heart Study. *BMJ*. 2008;337. DOI: 10.1136/bmj.a2338.

58. Christakis NA, Fowler JH. *Connected: How your friends' friends' friends affect everything you feel, think, and do.* Little Brown and Company. New York. 2009:51.

59. Christakis NA, Fowler JH. The spread of obesity in a large social network over 32 years. *N Eng J Med*. 2007;357:370-379.

60. Fowler JH, Christakis NA. Cooperative behavior cascades in human social networks. *PNAS*. 2010;107(12):5334-5338.

61. Waldinger R, Schultz M. *The Good Life: Lessons from the world's longest scientific study of happiness*. Simon & Schuster. New York, 2023.

62. Harvard Second Generation Study. Available at: https://www.adultdevelopmentstudy.org/. Accessed on March 18, 2023.

63. Waldinger R, Schultz M. *The Good Life: Lessons from the world's longest scientific study of happiness*. Simon & Schuster. New York, 2023:10.

64. Rohr R. *Breathing Under Water: Spirituality and the twelve steps*. Franciscan Media. Cincinnati, Ohio. 2021.

65. Rohr R. *Everything Belongs: The gift of contemplative prayer*. Crossroad Publishing Company. 2003.

66. Rohr R. *True Self, False Self*. (audiobook) Franciscan Media. Cincinnati, Ohio. 2010.

67. Star M. *Julian of Norwich: The Showings: Uncovering the face of the feminine in revelations of divine love*. Hamptons Roads Publishing. Newburyport, MA. 2022.

68. Bourgeault C. *The Wisdom Jesus: Transforming heart and mind—a new perspective of Christ and his message*. Shambhala Publishing. Berkeley, CA. 2008.

69. Rohr R. *The Wisdom Pattern: order, disorder, reorder*. Franciscan Media, Cincinnati, OH. 2020.

70. Strecher V. *Life on purpose: How living for what matters most changes everything*. Harper One. San Francisco. 2016.

71. Tolle E. The power of now. Yogi Impressions Books. Mumbai, India. 2006.

72. Center for Action and Contemplation. Daily Reflections. Discerning what is ours to do. August 2022. Available at: https://cac.org/daily-meditations/discerning-what-is-ours-to-do-weekly-summary-2022-08-27/. Accessed on March 18, 2023.

73. Merriam-Webster Dictionary (online). Available at: https://www.merriam-webster.com/. Accessed on March 18, 2023.

74. Center for Action and Contemplation. What is contemplation? Available at: https://cac.org/about/what-is-contemplation/. Accessed on March 18, 2023.

75. Keating T. *Open Mind, Open Heart,* 20th anniversary edition. Bloomsbury. London. 2006:175.

76. Contemplative Outreach. Centering Prayer. Available at: https://www.contemplativeoutreach.org/centering-prayer-method/. Accessed on March 18, 2023.

www.ingramcontent.com/pod-product-compliance
Lightning Source LLC
LaVergne TN
LVHW091552130126
829742LV00009B/205